Expectant Father's Handbook

A Modern Guide to Navigating Pregnancy

By

Terry A. Carreno

Content

DISCLAIMER

Introduction

Congratulations! You are embarking on the journey of fatherhood, and it's completely normal to have a mix of emotions right now – happiness, excitement, stress, nervousness, fear, or even a combination of them all. It might also feel overwhelming, and that's okay. Some men might not feel much at this point, and that's also perfectly fine.

The important thing is that you are here, willing to explore and understand what fatherhood means to you. Throughout this guide, our focus will be on helping you navigate the experience of being a dad, taking care of yourself and those around you, and becoming a confident and capable father. Some men become fathers through a deliberate and intentional process, having actively decided to become dads and taking the necessary steps to reach that goal. On the other hand, for some men, fatherhood comes as more of a surprise or even a shock.

When you first discover that fatherhood is on the horizon, you might not feel entirely prepared for it. However, it's essential not to let excessive worry consume you. Many men experience such feelings initially but often surprise themselves with how well they adapt to the role of a father. Learning and adjusting will largely come from finding your own path and trusting your instincts, which are likely more capable than you realize. Remember, no parent is perfect, and making mistakes is part of the learning process.

As a Dad, you'll discover that nature has equipped you for this journey, just as women are inherently prepared for motherhood. Fathers can be just as sensitive to a baby's cries as mothers are, and we can develop strong bonds with our children, even if they don't share our genes or live with us full-time. In fact, within hours of birth, we can recognize our babies by the touch of their hands, even when blindfolded. The key lies in investing time and effort, as these bonds can become as strong as iron.

No matter how enthusiastic you are about the prospect of becoming a father, there are likely many ways in which you might feel unprepared. It's possible that you don't feel financially ready for this responsibility, especially if you've been enjoying a carefree lifestyle and feel it has come too soon. The idea of taking on the responsibility of caring for a tiny human might also make you worry about potential restrictions or feeling tied down.

On an emotional level, you might not feel fully prepared. Uncertainty might exist regarding your relationship with the child's mother, or you could be experiencing difficulties with other important people in your life, including family members. Becoming a father often prompts us to reflect on our relationships with our own fathers and contemplate how we want to approach parenting.

These concerns and thoughts are entirely natural and common. It's essential to recognize that thousands of men have felt the same way when they became fathers, so you are not alone in these feelings. No matter who you are or what your life entails, it's crucial to recognize that you hold immense significance in the lives of your children, and your influence on them is profound. Your actions and choices, as well as what you choose not to do, will deeply impact how they learn and grow – from their academic achievements to their behavior, self-esteem, attitude towards risk, and the relationships they form with others. Essentially, you play a pivotal role in shaping the individuals they will become. It's essential not to underestimate the opportunity you have to make a positive difference in the world through your role as a father.

To assist you on your journey of fatherhood, we have created this guide to address the questions and concerns you are likely to have. We also provide information to direct you to the help and advice you might require along the way. Our hope is that this guide will aid you in one of the most significant and rewarding roles in the world – that of becoming a Dad!

This guide is crafted from the latest and most reliable research while also incorporating the insights of numerous fathers who have already undergone this journey. You don't have to follow it like a novel, reading from start to finish, although that option is available if you prefer. Instead, feel free to explore different chapters at your convenience, depending on what feels most relevant to you at any given time. Our primary aim is for you to find this guide helpful and beneficial to your experience.

Chapter 1

Accepting the New Role

Becoming a father is akin to embarking on one of life's grand adventures. Similar to the best journeys, there may be moments when you feel like you're navigating without a map. Fatherhood brings about profound changes within us, influencing our emotions, identity, and place in the world. It also fosters a deep connection that often becomes the essence of our existence: the bond with our children.

Experiencing doubts about whether you can excel at being a good father or uncertainty about your role is entirely normal. These feelings are part of how nature readies us for the transformations ahead. The process of 'becoming Dad' occurs gradually over months and years, extending beyond the instant when we first hold our child in our arms. Thus, fatherhood is an evolving journey, and each of us undergoes a unique experience, yet the emotional impact is universal and profound.

Dads during pregnancy experience a different path to parenthood compared to women, who physically carry the babies. However, this doesn't mean that the nine-month pregnancy period has no impact on men and leaves them untouched emotionally. Oxytocin, often referred to as the 'love' hormone, was traditionally thought to be essential only for women, particularly in inducing childbirth and facilitating breastfeeding.

Nonetheless, recent scientific research has revealed that oxytocin also holds significance for men, playing a central role in forming our relationships. Collaborating with other hormones like dopamine, the 'reward' hormone, oxytocin facilitates the establishment of bonds with our partners, children, and even friends. Additionally, testosterone, alongside these hormones, also influences your actions and emotions as a father, starting from before you even meet your child! During pregnancy, expectant mothers and fathers who live together exhibit remarkably similar levels of oxytocin. This phenomenon occurs because when we are in close and supportive relationships with others, our speech and movements tend to mirror theirs. Other forms of synchronization can also occur, such as our heart rate, body temperature, and blood pressure adjusting to similar levels. This oxytocin synchronization is akin to these harmonious connections.

The significance of this synchronization lies in the fact that oxytocin fosters increased empathy and cooperation among parents and makes them more open to the impending arrival of the baby. Particularly for fathers, it may reduce their focus on external rewards and encourage them to become more family-oriented. This priming effect prepares parents to work together as a team even before the baby is born. This synchronization could also explain why both fathers and mothers often engage in nesting behaviors before their children arrive. Creating physical space for the baby, like transforming a spare room into a nursery, and preparing with baby clothes, car seats, and other essentials is common. Moreover, fathers build a mental space by talking and singing to the baby bump, helping the unborn child recognize their voices. Fathers also imagine what the baby might look like and experience joy when feeling the baby kick or move in the mother's tummy. Ultrasound scans further allow fathers to emotionally connect with their unborn children. At this stage, fathers begin to form a bond with their babies even before their actual birth.

What type of father do you aspire to become?
The roles of women in early motherhood are firmly defined by the physical demands of pregnancy, childbirth, and breastfeeding. In contrast, as fathers, our roles can adapt rapidly in response to any changes in the social, economic, or physical environment that might affect our family's well-being. We have the ability to step up and provide whatever our children need the most.

In high-risk environments, fathers primarily focus on ensuring the baby's physical survival and health. In areas with food scarcity or war zones, fathering revolves around equipping the child with the necessary skills for economic survival. Once those fundamental needs are met, we can then turn our attention to supporting the child's social, cultural, and intellectual development.

In developed Western economies like the UK, much of our role as dads involves helping our children thrive economically and socially. This includes providing for their basic needs, imparting essential skills, guiding them, and supporting their education. The expectations placed on fathers have evolved significantly, and it's no longer enough to simply be the breadwinner. Nowadays, many fathers also want to actively participate in parenting while mothers pursue careers.

For many fathers, sharing all aspects of caregiving and earning becomes essential to manage the demands of modern family life. This can be challenging, especially for those who have limited family time due to work commitments. Like working mothers, most working fathers try to balance busy careers while actively being involved in raising their children. However, this balancing act can sometimes lead to feelings of guilt or the perception of underperforming both at work and at home.

Chapter 2

Taking care of yourself is of utmost importance.

In recent times, discussions surrounding mental health are prevalent everywhere. Social media platforms like Instagram and Facebook are filled with various advice on how to maintain good mental well-being. But how does all of this relate to becoming a father? Well, you are experiencing a significant life change, and it can be overwhelming. Fatherhood brings both joy and challenges that may increase stress, lead to conflicts, and leave you feeling off balance.

To cope effectively, it is essential to start by taking care of your physical health, such as staying physically active and eating healthily.

While getting sufficient sleep is crucial, it might be scarce during the early days of fatherhood. If you are accustomed to intense physical activities, consider adjusting your routine or engaging in gentler exercises that you and the mother can do together.

At times, you may feel exhausted and perhaps even isolated. It's vital to maintain contact with the outside world, even if it means going for short walks or runs, spending time in the garden or park, talking to friends, and pursuing your interests.

Engage in regular self-check-ins to assess how you are feeling.

Consider using apps like the notes app on your phone to keep a record of your experiences, both positive and challenging. You can even score your mood on a scale from one to five. By doing so, you can identify patterns or triggers that may impact your well-being negatively. This self-reflection will help you discover ways to maintain your emotional well-being and keep yourself feeling positive and healthy.

Learning to relax

It is an essential skill that benefits both mothers and fathers, as you might have already noticed in childbirth classes. If you decide to be present at the birth, employing calm, deep breathing techniques can help manage anxiety, create a serene atmosphere, and support labor progression.

Breathing exercises aren't only valuable for fathers during childbirth; they are beneficial in various situations as your children grow older. As a father, learning to quickly relax can aid in staying composed. This self-awareness allows you to better manage frustrations with your partner, your child, and even yourself.

To induce relaxation, try taking a long, deep breath and exhale slowly, releasing stress and tension. A useful technique involves expanding your stomach when inhaling and contracting it during exhalation, contrary to the usual breathing pattern. This method significantly calms your brain, body, and mind.

You may want to explore additional relaxation techniques like meditation, mindfulness, or yoga exercises, as many fathers find them beneficial and swear by their positive effects.

Remember, you're not alone in this journey of fatherhood.

Men have been embracing fatherhood since the beginning of human life, whether as biological fathers, stepfathers, or adoptive fathers. While each father's path is unique, the experience of becoming a dad is universal, connecting millions of fathers worldwide. Knowing this can offer reassurance, as there are countless other fathers to learn from and connect with.

As a father, you will need to connect and maintain connections with various people in your child's life. Building a strong, positive co-parenting relationship with your child's mother, regardless of your relationship status, should be a priority. Remember that fatherhood extends beyond just you and your child's mother; it involves various individuals who play important roles in your child's life.

Preparing for fatherhood through fitness

Becoming a dad introduces new pressures and responsibilities that may limit the time available for staying fit. However, it's crucial to establish a routine of regular exercise, especially if you haven't been doing so already. Engaging in physical activity will help you better cope with the fatigue and stress that often accompany the arrival of a new baby.

Being a fit dad also has a long-term impact on your children's exercise habits, from infancy to adolescence. In fact, fathers who regularly engage in physical exercise play a significant role in predicting their teenagers' activity levels, whether they are girls or boys.

Incorporating exercise into your daily life doesn't have to be complicated or expensive, even if you're busy. There are plenty of low-cost and straightforward exercises you can do, from stair climbing and walking to skipping, that can easily be integrated into your daily routine.

Chapter 3

Assisting the biological mother of your baby.

Transitioning into motherhood can be quite a challenge. Despite pregnancy, birth, and breastfeeding being natural parts of life, it's essential to recognize that human reproduction is a remarkable miracle. Alongside your journey to fatherhood, someone else is experiencing an almost unbelievable physical and emotional transformation.

These changes are primarily due to hormonal shifts, their bodies adapting to accommodate the growing baby, and the added responsibilities of nourishing and caring for the child. As you can imagine, these aspects combine to become a significant undertaking.

While some women seem to handle this transformation with ease, others may find it more difficult, and for some, it can be an outright struggle. However, most, if not all, cope better when the people closest to them, including fathers like us, provide them with both physical comfort and emotional support.

Caring for her physical well-being

Fathers-to-be can play a vital role in supporting their partner's physical health during and after pregnancy. Here are five essential ways to provide assistance:

- Encourage her to rest, particularly during the challenging initial 12 weeks of pregnancy, which is the period when she is most vulnerable to miscarriage.
- Engage in exercise together. Children are more likely to adopt exercise habits if

they see their father doing so. By cultivating healthy exercise routines now, you can set a positive example for your children and support your partner's well-being too.

- Quit smoking. Remember that second-hand smoke can be harmful to both her and the baby. If she is a smoker, your efforts to reduce or quit smoking can inspire her to do the same.
- Limit alcohol and caffeine intake. Reducing your consumption of alcohol and caffeine can help prevent iron absorption issues and encourage her to do the same.
- Assist her in maintaining a balanced diet. Taking charge of preparing healthy meals can be beneficial, especially if she experiences morning sickness. Foods

rich in iron, such as red meat, wholemeal bread, lentils, beans, broccoli, dried apricots, figs, and iron-fortified breakfast cereals, can help prevent anemia. Ensure she also consumes enough calcium from sources like milk, yogurt, cheese, tofu, broccoli, and dried fruit. Fiber-rich foods like wholemeal bran can prevent constipation and piles. If she experiences indigestion or heartburn, encourage her to have small meals, sit upright while eating, and avoid eating or drinking a few hours before bedtime.

Women's emotional journey
Research indicates that up to one in five women experience depression or anxiety during pregnancy or the first year after childbirth. Many of them undergo stress, loss of

confidence, and reduced self-esteem. Before the baby's arrival, they may feel upset about their body changes and have concerns about the birthing process and the baby's health. After labor and delivery, they require time to recover, and if they are breastfeeding, establishing and maintaining a close bond around feeding can be physically and emotionally draining.

Similar to fathers-to-be, women also face significant adjustments when they become mothers. The societal notion that women are "natural" parents can lead many mothers to feel inadequate compared to the idealized vision of motherhood. Peer support from other moms and guidance from professionals like midwives and health visitors, who often have personal experience as mothers, can help women navigate the changes they are undergoing and their associated emotions.

We, as fathers, have a crucial role to play too. By creating a safe space for mothers to express their thoughts and fears, offering understanding and support, reassuring them of their greatness and love, and helping them feel positive about their appearance, we contribute to their well-being.

Dealing with mood swings

Some men may find expectant mothers' emotions to be unpredictable. They might experience a mix of happiness, shock, excitement, and worry simultaneously. Women can become hypersensitive and react strongly to what others perceive as minor issues, or they may be upset or angry about seemingly insignificant matters. Forgetfulness and difficulty concentrating are also common.

It is essential to understand that her hormones will stabilize after the initial few months. Your role is not to solve her feelings but to listen, empathize, and show love. Calming breathing exercises can help during stressful times, and it's important to avoid arguing at such moments. Open communication and talking about feelings can be beneficial.

Since both of you are undergoing significant changes, seeking outside help may be necessary at times. Feelings of anger, sadness, loneliness, or fear can be addressed through conversations with others who have experienced similar situations. Speaking with other fathers, friends who are already dads, or seeking support from Dads' groups can provide valuable insights and help process emotions.

Be cautious about taking on significant new projects at work because you already have an important one at home: becoming a Dad! It's also essential not to become overly ambitious with home projects. Sometimes, in anticipation of a baby's arrival, our nesting instincts may lead us to tackle substantial DIY tasks like reorganizing and redecorating rooms or even moving to a new house. However, it's worth considering that babies need very little space until they start walking, and they don't have preferences for wall colors. The most crucial focus should be on nurturing your relationships with each other and with the baby. Perhaps the house-related tasks can wait until the baby is a bit older?

Dealing with sleep problems

Expectant mothers may experience difficulty getting enough sleep even before birth. If you live together, her sleeplessness may also affect your rest. Frequent trips to the bathroom or discomfort in finding a comfortable sleeping position can be contributing factors. As a result, both of you may feel tired and irritable during the day.

People around you may advise you to get used to this sleep disruption since there will likely be plenty of broken sleep when the baby arrives. Unfortunately, they are correct. Some women find it more comfortable to sleep with a pillow or other support, so it's worth exploring different solutions to promote better rest during pregnancy. Support her even if her pregnancy is affecting your sleep routine, as she is carrying your baby and has no choice but to endure the physical changes. Encourage her to rest, especially in the first 12 weeks of pregnancy, when she is at a higher risk of miscarriage.

Preparing for the birth

During the journey from conception to childbirth, both Mum and you will attend various midwife appointments, scans, and tests leading up to the baby's arrival. Along the way, important decisions must be made, such as choosing where to have the baby, discussing preferences for pain relief, and considering options like water birth. While these choices primarily belong to Mum, they also depend on what options are available in your local area.

As a birth partner, your role is to assist Mum in obtaining the necessary information to make informed decisions and to support her in whatever choices she makes. Attending antenatal classes, asking questions to midwives, and referring to reliable websites can help both of you gain a better understanding of what feels right for your unique situation.

Occasionally, even the best-laid plans may face setbacks, and you may need to adapt your expectations about pregnancy and birth. In such instances, it's crucial to maintain open conversations with Mum, offer support during the adjustment period, and discuss any concerns that may arise. Seek information together and consider seeking support from trusted networks or websites if needed. Don't hesitate to inquire further if you feel you need more information than what you've been provided.

In rare situations, healthcare professionals may deliver concerning news about the baby, putting both of you in a position to decide whether to terminate the pregnancy or not. During such challenging times, it's essential to give each other space to process and discuss the situation. Focus on supporting one another, share your feelings with trusted family and friends, and ask any necessary questions to medical professionals. Specialist organizations and bereavement counseling can also be valuable resources during these difficult times.

Your guide to contractions

At some point, Mum may experience contractions. These are typically known as Braxton Hicks contractions (named after the 19th-century doctor who discovered them). They serve as a practice run for the body to get accustomed to the sensation of labor. Braxton Hicks contractions last for a few seconds, causing a strong tightening sensation across the belly and sometimes in the back and legs, before subsiding. Initially, they might feel uncomfortable or even scary, but they differ from "real" labor contractions as they don't establish a regular rhythm. On the other hand, true labor involves slow, consistent contractions that gradually intensify, often accompanied by pain in the lower legs, back, and abdomen. If her water has not broken, there is no need to contact the midwife until contractions are about ten minutes apart.

If she experiences Braxton Hicks contractions, movement can be beneficial. Encourage her to change positions or try deep breathing exercises while they occur. Sometimes, engaging in sexual activity might trigger

Braxton Hicks contractions, but rest assured that it does not lead to premature birth or endanger the baby.

Being a birth partner

Many men may feel like a spare part when entering the labor ward, and unfortunately, they often receive little guidance on their role. Here's our recommendation to clarify your role as a birth partner. While you might have seen birth scenes on TV where the mother is lying on a hospital bed with her knees up and legs open, it's important to note that alternative positions and staying upright can make the process less painful for her and potentially speed up labor.

During the first stage of labor (opening contractions), she has various options for positions. She could lean on the wall, a chair, or hold onto you while rocking her pelvis. Kneeling up while holding onto you or kneeling down on all fours and rocking might be comfortable for her. Sitting upright on a large ball or getting into a warm bath or birth pool could also be favorable options.

When it's time for the second stage of labor (pushing), staying upright can aid in a quicker delivery. Being upright widens her pelvis, allowing the baby to descend more easily. For instance, she could kneel on the floor and hold onto the bed or kneel on the bed and hold onto you.

As the birth partner, you can serve as the mother's support during labor, whether it feels fun, a bit scary, or overwhelming. Consider discussing your role with the midwife beforehand to feel more confident and prepared for the experience.

Dilation: What is it and why is it important?

During labor, you may hear healthcare professionals discussing dilation. This refers to the mother's cervix, which is the neck of her womb. Throughout pregnancy, the cervix remains closed, and during labor, it needs to open to allow the baby to be born. Contractions gradually open the cervix little by little. The midwife will check its level of dilation during labor, and once it reaches 10cm, it is considered fully open (or 'dilated'), signaling that it's time for her to begin pushing the baby out.

Dilation of the cervix is a crucial marker for monitoring the progress of labor, and midwives closely observe this aspect. It's worth noting that the birthing process can be invasive for women, and it's essential to remind expectant mothers that they don't have to undergo a vaginal examination if they prefer not to. As her birth partner, you can advocate for her and ensure her wishes are respected and heard.

The power of breathing

Proper breathing is essential for both the mother and baby during labor, as it can make the birthing experience feel more controlled and less panicked. It can help reduce the pain experienced during labor and ensure that both receive sufficient oxygen. Practicing deep breathing techniques in advance can be immensely beneficial for her, and it will prepare you to support her during labor.

When a woman is in labor, her uterine muscles contract and tighten more intensely. If she feels tense or scared, other muscles in her body may also tighten, leading to increased pain during labor. Additionally, panic can cause her breathing to become shallow and fast, potentially affecting oxygen intake for both mother and baby.

To prevent these issues, many women practice relaxation and deep breathing exercises with their partners before labor. This helps foster a sense of calmness during the birthing process. You can practice breathing together in the weeks leading up to labor, making it more second nature when you are in the birthing room – see Box 6: How to do breathing practice.

Recovery after birth

The birthing process can be physically demanding and messy. New mothers may experience bruising and swelling. If she had a vaginal birth, there might have been an episiotomy (a surgical cut) or a tear to facilitate the baby's head's emergence, resulting in stitches. The recovery process will vary from woman to woman, and she will need time to heal and rest after giving birth.

Preparing for Breastfeeding

When your baby is born, even if you're unable to provide milk from your body, you can still play a crucial role in supporting their feeding journey. Creating a calm environment for both Mum and the baby while she tries to breastfeed can be challenging, but your encouragement can make all the difference.

Whether or not she plans to breastfeed for an extended period, it's worth her trying it for the first few days because the initial milk her body produces is incredibly special. Known as 'colostrum,' it's the perfect first food for your baby, packed with all the essential nutrients they need. Colostrum not only provides protection against germs but is also easily digestible for their tiny tummy, helps prevent jaundice (a condition causing a baby's skin to turn yellow), and aids in their first bowel movement.

An essential aspect of feeding is 'responsive feeding.' This involves Mum establishing eye-to-eye contact with the baby and delivering food slowly. Feeding becomes like a conversation, an interactive back-and-forth experience with moments of pausing before continuing. It's crucial to maintain a calm and peaceful atmosphere during feeding, in a quiet place where everyone involved can relax and cherish this significant bonding time.

As your baby progresses to other forms of feeding, the responsibility can be shared. For now, your role is to make feeding a pleasurable experience for everyone. After feeding is finished, Mum might hand the baby over to you, indicating that feeding time is over for the moment. You may become an expert at "burping," gently rubbing your baby's back after feeding and helping them settle down to sleep.

Chapter 4

The Well-being of Your Relationship

Creating Time for Open Communication

Becoming parents can evoke a range of emotions and thoughts for both you and your partner, from excitement to worry. It's completely normal. To maintain closeness during this time, set aside a regular moment to talk and truly listen to each other. Communication might be different and more challenging now, given the additional responsibilities, so try using the "Speaker/Listener" technique. Take turns being the "Speaker" for one minute, then switch to become the "Listener." Listen actively without interruptions, disagreements, or offering solutions. You can even pass a metaphorical "speaking baton" between you to make it a bit more playful. It's beneficial to practice this technique regularly, and over time, it will become a natural part of your communication style. Utilize this approach to check in with each other once your baby arrives.

Deciding on Roles and Responsibilities

Traditional gender roles might influence some people's beliefs about the roles of fathers and mothers in the family. However, it's essential to recognize that these roles can be flexible and adaptable to your unique situation. Some may assume that fathers should be the primary breadwinners and mothers should be "stay at home Mums" responsible for caregiving. However, in non-traditional families, like gay couples, similar assumptions may arise even if the roles don't align with traditional gender norms.

Discussing "who does what" in your relationship, particularly concerning childcare and household tasks, is crucial. Research indicates that parent-couples tend to be happier and more connected when they share earning, caring, and domestic responsibilities. Rather than making assumptions based on stereotypes, it's essential to have clear and agreed-upon divisions of tasks. Avoid assumptions like "she's at home with the baby, so she'll do most of the housework" or "he'll handle all the DIY because he's a man and men enjoy that kind of thing." Open communication and shared decision-making are key to maintaining a happy and balanced partnership.

Resolving Disagreements

Parenting comes with a variety of challenges, and there are multiple ways to approach them. How you handle tasks like feeding, burping, settling, and sleeping for your child may differ from your partner's approach. It's essential to have regular discussions to settle any disagreements that may arise. As a Dad, if you want an equal role in these conversations, you need to put in the effort and gain practical experience rather than relying solely on theory. Emulate what mothers have been doing for a long time: ask questions, seek knowledge, and read blogs about child-rearing. Take the initiative, do the work, and gain confidence in your parenting abilities. Encourage Mum to step back at times, making space for you to actively engage as a father. This is especially important if you find yourself surrounded by people who believe that mothers always know best.

Arguing Constructively

Research reveals that nearly nine out of ten first-time parents argue more than before the child was born. This increase in arguments is normal as you both navigate through significant changes and numerous discussions. The key is to learn how to argue constructively, ensuring that both partners feel heard and understood.

Here are some top tips for constructive arguing:

- Start discussions with positive comments instead of harsh criticism to avoid defensiveness.
- Avoid making generalizations and stick to specific facts.

- Expand your emotional expressions beyond anger, including sadness, fear, and disappointment.
- If you need a break during heated discussions, communicate it as a "time out" to return to the conversation later.
- Try to resolve conflicts before bedtime and be the one to extend an olive branch.

Coping with Sleep Deprivation

Sleeplessness in babies is a common challenge in early parenthood, leaving parents tired and grumpy. While it may be challenging, the moments during nighttime awakenings with your baby can also be precious and intimate. Providing comfort and care during these times can strengthen your bond with your child. Some babies may have more difficulty sleeping than others, and in such cases, it's crucial to share the responsibility and support each other.

Dealing with Grandparents

All grandparents will have their own thoughts and opinions about your baby and how you should raise them. Some may want to be actively involved, while others might take a step back. Sometimes, they could be pushy, insisting on specific parenting approaches. However, as parents, it's essential for you and Mum to communicate your needs and preferences to them. If necessary, don't hesitate to ask them to give you space and allow you to make decisions about parenting. It's your right to decide what kind of parents you want to be, not theirs.

Over-enthusiastic extended family members can sometimes overshadow fathers in decision-making, with mothers inadvertently allowing it to happen. To avoid this, have open discussions with your partner about maintaining a consistent message and shared responsibilities.

Navigating Changes in Your Sex Life

Becoming parents can impact your sex life, but it doesn't have to be the end of intimacy and connection. Pregnancy, childbirth, recovery, and breastfeeding can lead to changes in a woman's sexual desires, with some experiencing increased attraction and intimacy, while others may feel differently. All of these responses are normal and natural.

Sex is generally safe during pregnancy, though you may need to explore different positions for comfort as her body changes. Engaging in sexual activity won't cause a miscarriage. It's a natural part of life and should be approached with understanding and communication. Late in pregnancy, having an orgasm might trigger practice contractions, but it won't induce labor. However, if there's any heavy bleeding, it's best to consult a midwife or doctor before engaging in sexual activity.

After childbirth, the timing of resuming sexual activity varies from one person to another, and it's essential to be patient and understanding. Many new mothers prefer to wait at least a month or two due to soreness and exhaustion. Pressure should not be put on the mother to start again before she feels comfortable. Using condoms for the first six weeks after birth is recommended to prevent infections during the healing process.

It's normal for fathers to have concerns about hurting their partner during sex or feeling rejected due to reduced intimacy. It's essential to communicate with your partner, express your support and attraction, and understand her need to recover. Let her know that you're looking forward to intimacy again, but there's no rush, and her comfort and well-being are the priority.

Chapter 5

Getting acquainted with your baby

Engage with your unborn baby by talking to the bump, as babies can listen and learn even while in the womb. Initially, it might feel unusual, but this practice can become a meaningful habit. Though they won't comprehend the words, they will become accustomed to the comforting sound of your voice and its rhythms.

Speak to the bump at a normal volume, as if having a casual chat, without the need to shout or whisper. You can even read to them, introducing them to the sounds they will encounter in their everyday life once they're born. This inclusion helps them understand that you, their Dad, are an essential part of their world.

Playing soothing music during pregnancy not only benefits the mother's well-being but also has a positive impact on the unborn child's brain development. As the baby's brain develops, they start reacting to the sounds they hear. Lullabies, in particular, can have a calming effect on the baby, leading to stillness or reduced movements. Research even suggests that babies may recognize music they heard in the womb after birth.

When playing music, keep the volume low to maintain a calm environment for your baby. Pay attention to their movements, as they might indicate a reaction to the noise level. Singing to your baby, regardless of your vocal abilities, can also foster early bonding and prove helpful in soothing them after birth by singing familiar songs.

From anticipation to reality

Once the baby is born, the relationship you've been imagining comes to life. Embracing skin-to-skin contact with your newborn is a simple yet significant step both you and Mum can take to welcome them into the world. This practice offers benefits to everyone involved:

For the baby, it reduces stress and helps regulate their breathing and temperature.

For Mums, it fosters a close bond with the baby and aids in getting in sync for breastfeeding.

For Dads, it activates hormones associated with love and happiness, like oxytocin and serotonin, while reducing testosterone levels, fostering closeness and readiness to care for the baby.

Typically, midwives place the baby directly on Mum's chest after a normal delivery, so as a Dad, you might need to wait your turn. This might make you feel like a "secondary" parent at this moment, but it's natural as Mum has been through a significant experience and is designed to initiate breastfeeding. Witnessing her meet and connect with the tiny miracle she delivered is a beautiful experience.

However, be prepared for when it's your turn, as there might be situations where you get to hold the baby first, especially if Mum has a C-section or needs stitches. Wear clothing that allows easy access, like a shirt with front buttons, so you can have skin-to-skin contact with your baby, placing them close to your heart and covering both of you with a soft blanket.

This special moment of holding your baby skin-to-skin can be incredibly precious and life-changing, so be fully present and immerse yourself in the experience instead of getting distracted by taking pictures.

Remember, skin-to-skin contact isn't limited to the first day of your baby's life. You can continue doing it for months, as it is a wonderful way to deeply connect with your newborn and provide comfort when they are tired or fussy.

In the early days, biological mothers had a natural advantage as caregivers due to their unique role in giving birth and the neurochemicals involved in labor and breastfeeding. Oxytocin and beta-endorphin, which play a crucial role in labor and bonding, help them form a connection with the baby, although it may still take some time for some mothers to feel that bond.

As fathers, we rely on physical and verbal interactions with the baby to foster our bond since we don't have the biological advantage that mothers do. However, this can be challenging, especially when the baby seeks comfort from the mother most of the time, particularly during breastfeeding, when only she can provide food. Additionally, newborns are not very interactive, and they don't smile or respond to jokes, making it easy for us to feel detached.

The continuous cycle of changing diapers, hunger cries, and disrupted sleep can exacerbate these feelings. As the baby seeks comfort from and is soothed by the mother, we might feel increasingly down and left out.

Play Time

The idea that fathers have a special role as playmates for our babies may sound like a cliché, but research indicates that there's truth to this notion. As babies become more interactive, many of us find it easier to relate to them and enjoy their company. Simple playful gestures like making silly faces or blowing raspberries on their tummy can elicit smiles and laughter from our babies.

Play often comes naturally and instinctively, and as long as we prioritize our baby's safety and enjoyment, we'll likely find ourselves inventing fun little activities. While you don't need an array of toys, having a few familiar items can be helpful in soothing and entertaining them. Babies can delight in playing with water (always under supervision), leaves, boxes, or cut-up pieces of fabric.

As babies grow into toddlers, we may engage in more boisterous "rough and tumble" play, involving physical activities that make them giggle and belly laugh. Activities like lifting them into the air, tickling, running around, and rolling together can be great fun. Even babies between six to twelve months can enjoy lighter versions of such play, like lifting them up or bouncing them on our knees, rolling, climbing, and tumbling over people. Making repetitive noises, such as pretending they are a plane, can add to the enjoyment.

Balancing work and family life

This can be a challenge for us fathers, especially when we feel the pressure to suppress our emotions and prioritize work over our roles as dads. It's important for our employers to be aware of our impending fatherhood, and while taking paternity leave is a step in the right direction, it may not fully convey the significant change happening in our lives.

Unfortunately, some employers may not be as understanding about our parental responsibilities, particularly for male employees. Despite offering generous maternity benefits for female staff, they may be less supportive when it comes to fathers seeking similar arrangements. This can make it daunting for us to advocate for a better work-life balance, especially if we are the main breadwinners or work in environments with a traditional macho culture that values long office hours above family commitments.

In some cases, it may be necessary to seek a new job that aligns better with our desire for work-life balance. However, it's also possible that by opening up about our domestic lives and challenging outdated norms, we can contribute to creating a more accepting workplace. We might be the trailblazers, advocating for modern fatherhood, where being present for our families is as valued as our commitment to work.

Ultimately, the decision of whether to challenge the status quo or seek a more family-friendly work environment depends on individual circumstances. It involves weighing potential risks, such as being viewed as less committed by our employers, against the benefits of being seen as a caring family man who values both work and family life. If we want to actively participate in our child's life without feeling apologetic, it's essential to consider the options and make a choice that aligns with our priorities.

Chapter 6

Facing Challenges and need Support

Becoming a father can be an exhausting and stressful experience. While most dads manage to handle it, some may find it challenging to cope with the changes that come with having a child. People generally recognize the physical and emotional transformations that mothers go through, but it's essential to acknowledge that fathers are impacted by these changes too.

Welcoming a new baby can bring about significant shifts for both mothers and fathers, and not all of these changes are easy to adapt to. It's common to feel frustrated with less time and energy, or to experience feelings of low mood, being overwhelmed, or having racing thoughts. Having a baby represents a major life change, and each father processes this change differently. The reasons why some dads are affected more than others can be a combination of factors, including hormonal changes, the stress of caring for a newborn, adjustments to lifestyle, and individual upbringing and experiences.

For some dads, the arrival of a baby can affect their mental health, while others may not experience the same impact. Mental health encompasses the well-being of our thoughts, feelings, and reactions. It's essential to remember that mental health is not solely about poor mental health; it also involves maintaining good mental health through positive actions, which can help us cope better when facing challenging times in life. It's crucial to keep in mind that the majority of fathers do not experience mental health issues. However, this doesn't mean you are expected to feel fantastic or completely fine every single day. It's entirely normal to have moments of feeling a bit low or flat after welcoming a new baby.

A temporary low mood is common and typically improves over a short period. Experiencing such emotions doesn't make you a bad dad, nor does it indicate a lack of love for your baby. It merely suggests that you are navigating a significant life transition. Similar to your physical health, your mental well-being may require some extra attention and care. Prioritizing your mental health will lead to an improved quality of life and positively impact your family.

It's essential to embrace who you are as a father. Every dad is unique, and the role of being a dad can be both challenging and rewarding. You might have skills in making your kids laugh or creating enjoyable family adventures. Additionally, you might excel at cooking and teaching them new things. Recognize that there are many aspects that make you a great dad. Taking care of yourself can have a positive impact on your mood. Sometimes, feeling low can be a signal from our bodies that we need to focus more on our well-being. It's important to confide in someone you trust about your low or bad days, whether it's your partner, family members, or friends. Open communication is essential, as your loved ones cannot support you effectively if they are unaware of how you're feeling.

Friends and family can offer practical assistance to give you some space and relieve some of the pressure on you and your partner. However, not everyone may have someone they feel comfortable talking to. It's possible that the people we want to talk to may not fully understand our experiences, especially if they haven't been fathers themselves. To address this, some fathers have formed peer support groups where they can share their experiences with others in the same stage of life. Additionally, some dads have created websites, blogs, and social media platforms to share their journey of becoming a father.

Ultimately, fathers can relate to each other's struggles and challenges in coping with fatherhood better than anyone else. By connecting with other dads, you can find understanding, support, and valuable insights to navigate this transformative phase of life. Seeking support as a father may not always be easy, especially if you feel responsible for providing support to your family. However, just like with physical health, there are limits to what we can handle alone when it comes to our mental well-being. Getting support early is crucial, and it's essential to talk to a healthcare professional about your feelings and struggles.

You can choose to talk directly to a healthcare professional or confide in your partner, family member, or a trusted friend first. Healthcare workers, such as your GP, are trained to identify mental health issues and can guide you to the appropriate support. They will keep your discussions confidential unless there's a risk to yourself or others, in which case they will inform you about their actions.

During a GP appointment, your doctor will inquire about your mood and overall health to assess both your mental and physical well-being and identify potential causes of your symptoms. It may be helpful to jot down your symptoms before the appointment to ensure you communicate everything effectively. Your GP will work with you to develop a plan for the best support moving forward, even if an immediate diagnosis is not possible.

In addition to professional support, peer support groups and online communities can offer valuable assistance. You might be surprised to find that many other fathers are experiencing similar feelings and symptoms. Connecting with other dads facing similar challenges allows you to share ideas, resources, and personal stories. Listening to other fathers' journeys through fatherhood can provide you with a sense of validation and offer ideas for coping with your own experiences.